Aloe Vera –

Nature's Secret

Things you never knew about Aloe Vera and its benefits

AMARPREET SINGH

Publisher - The Thought Flame

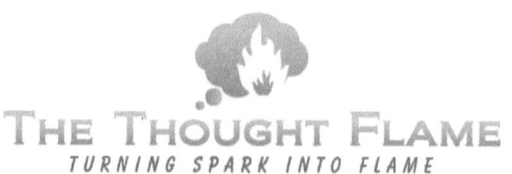

THE THOUGHT FLAME
TURNING SPARK INTO FLAME

info@thethoughtflame.com

www.thethoughtflame.com

Table of Contents

Introduction

In life it is damn near impossible to avoid getting hurt. At some point or another you will end up with a few injuries, some bumps, scraps, blisters, burns or cuts. That is life. However, there are many of us that have our own special family "recipes" to help cure almost any kind of scrape or cut on your body and that seems to be the miracle cure for almost any ailment. In my family that "cure" was Aloe Vera.

My great-grandmother was the one who used to administer Aloe Vera to nearly every member of her family. Even to this day I could still remember her two large Aloe Vera plants sitting on the windowsill looking as if they had been used one too many times.

It is within the plant itself that the true wonder and miracle of its healing abilities lie and to access this perfect remedy that seems to have the ability to heal almost any skin ailment, all that you need to do is cut off a leaf right at its base. Don't worry, its own healing properties will allow it to heal its own wounds and still remain a vibrant green color for many days to come.

Due to its magical healing properties Aloe is properly used for many different reasons and can even be found in many common items such as hair shampoo, burn ointments and even sunburn lotion. It is so popular in fact that even the United States government used it to help treat radiation burns in the past.

If you have never really heard of the Aloe Vera plant , then you are in luck. In this eBook you will learn about the famous history of this plant, what the health benefits are of using this plant and 25 different ways that you can use Aloe Vera to promote healing. With this eBook you will learn everything there is to learn about Aloe Vera so that you can harness the healing potential of this extraordinary plant.

So, what are you waiting for? Let's get started.

Chapter One: The Wonderful History of Aloe Vera

While Aloe Vera is no longer able to be found in the wild, it is one of the most abundant and common plants you will find in many households today. This is all thanks to the growing advances in technology, the Internet and the power of advertisement.

When researchers began examining this magical plant closely, there was many theories and evidence that could be found on it. To start the Aloe Vera plant, researchers believe, first originated somewhere in the driest and most desolate corners of both Madagascar and Africa. However, it didn't take long for this plant to escape the confines of these dry places on the planet when humans found that it had healing properties.

Because of man's curiosity over the plant and the realization that it had incredible healing properties, Aloe Vera has become one of the most highly cultivated plants on the planet today and it is one of the ones that you will find in most households. You can find this planet in almost every country such as Mexico, the United States, Japan, Russia and China.

What is even more amazing is that the Aloe Vera plants has been documented as being used for a variety of medicinal properties dating as far back as 3,500 years ago where the tombs of Pharaohs had paintings of this plant scribed all over the walls. Researchers have found that the plant dates back as far as Biblical times when the first appearance of the plant in record were seen on a clay tablet dating back to the Mesopotamian era, around 2,100 B.C.

Throughout history you can find descriptive records of how the Aloe Vera plant was used and how it was practically worshipped by many people across the world. Around 70 A.D researchers were able to find detailed records of how the people when used Aloe Vera to treat a variety of wounds and ailments such as hemorrhoids and hair loss.

During the time of the civil war archeologists were able to find that many cavalrymen had created a special "elixir" made with Aloe, some hemp pulp and a few drops of palm wine. Many man called it an elixir because they truly believed that the drink had the ability to make sure that the men would be able to live through battle and many even believed it would give them courage.

There are many times throughout history where you can see for yourself how this plant was used by the people living during that time period, what people thought of the plant's magical healing properties and how doctors of that time were able to help relieve patients of certain ailments. The Aloe plant popularly pops up throughout history, that being one of the main causes it continues to be one of the most researched plants today.

Even throughout history we can see that people from different time periods used the plant for a variety of reasons. Some of these reasons could have included healing cuts and wounds, to help improve digestion, to help relieve joint and muscle discomfort, to help sooth irritated skin and to help relieve stomach pain. What is even more surprising is that many people use the plant for the same reasons the people did in the past. Even over thousands of years this plant has not changed much.

There is really only one main conclusion that we can draw from Aloe Vera's long and detailed history: It is good for pretty much everything.

Chapter Two: The Wonderful Health Benefits of Using Aloe

When you take a step back and truly admire the Aloe Vera plant for what it is, you will quickly realize that it is full of nutritional benefits. Every person who uses this plant will quickly attest to what it does to their body and often have their own unique ways in which they use Aloe on a daily basis. As for myself I usually make a thick paste with fresh Aloe to help treat my eczema when I have a severe outbreak. I'll tell you what, it works better than Hydrocortisone ever did.

With the many different ways that you can use Aloe Vera, there are just as many different ways in which this plant can help you benefit health wise. In this chapter you will learn about the top ten health benefits of using this plant so that you may see how it will help you and your body the longer that you use it.

1. Aloe Vera Can Help With Your Digestion

While many people today seem to have the iron stomachs of a coz, there are some of us who have been unfortunately prone to various digestion issues. Whether you are suffering from irritable bowel syndrome, have just had your gallbladder removed or have just had a gastropexy, ingesting Aloe Vera can help ease some of the symptoms that you may be suffering from.

Having a digestive tract that just functions normally is a good sign that you are healthy, both inside and out. Using Aloe Vera can help make sure that your digestive tract remains as healthy as possible by helping to regulate your digestive tract and helping you to overcome nasty bouts of diarrhea or constipation.

2. Aloe Can Be Especially Beneficial For Your Heart

Heart disease is one of the main illness killing people in the United States today. It is so bad that more people are dying from heart disease every year than cancer alone. With high numbers like this, wouldn't you want to do everything in your power to help take care of your heart? By using Aloe Vera, now you can do exactly that.

For many years that have been a variety of studies conducted to see exactly how aloe benefits the heart and researchers found that when aloe is injected straight into the blood stream it helps to improve oxygenation in the blood, lowering the chances of a person developing high cholesterol in his or her lifetime and by lowering the risk of heart disease. With studies like this being conducted on a daily basis, it is still surprising why many people have not considered using Aloe to help keep their heart healthy.

3. It Can Help Give Your Immune System An Extra Boost

Did you know that every tiny thing that you stress about on a daily basis can have a negative effect on your immune system? Just think about. Have you ever noticed how many college students are sick as dogs right before they have to take their semester finals?

Well, when you use Aloe and ingest it whether it be in the form of a juice or a pulp, you can help give your immune system the extra boost that it sometimes needs. Researchers have found that Aloe Vera contains a high level of anti-oxidants, making it an excellent immune system enhancer. It also contains microscopic compounds known as polysaccharides, which have shown to stimulate the production and effectiveness of white blood cells in your body as they attack bacteria and viruses that wish to do your body harm.

Not only will Aloe help make sure that you avoid catching a sickness every time your nerves are shot, but it can help get you over a sickness faster than any medication on the market today.

4. Aloe Has A High Concentration Of Important Vitamins and Minerals That You Need On A Daily Basis

As we age we don't worry about taking in as many vitamins and minerals as we should be. That is because we are too busy worrying about other things such as paying our bills on time and making sure that our children are being taken care of properly.

There are a number of vitamins and minerals that we need to make sure we take insuch as Vitamins A, C, K, D, B1,B2, B3, Folic Acid and Biotin. These vitamins and minerals are essential for our bodies to be in a constant state of homeostasis and if we do not take them in every single day, we risk doing damage to our bodies in the long run.

By taking Aloe Vera in every day, you get all the vitamins and minerals that you need just from the plant itself as well as other important minerals such as Zinc, Potassium, Iron, Calcium, Magnesium, Manganese, Sodium, Copper, Selenium and Chromium.

5. Aloe Can Help You Lose Weight

Now, I know that I am not the only person that has suffer with weight most of their life and I know that I will certainly not be the last. The main issue about having problem losing weight or keeping it off is that many people are not taking in the essential vitamins, calories, minerals or water that they need to take. Some people may even have issues with their digestive tracks, which can also have a negative effect on a person's weight.

By using Aloe you give yourself the opportunity to help improve your body's digestion, which in turn will help to detoxify your body and allow you to lose weight more naturally and efficiently. Aloe will also give your body the energy it needs to lose weight.

6. Aloe Is Extremely Good For Your Skin

Nine times out of ten you have probably heard of Aloe by seeing plastered all over shampoos and lotion bottles. You may have even heard a couple claims to how effective Aloe is to help a person maintain healthy and young-looking skin. In fact Aloe is one of the key components used in many beauty care products today and is one of the ingredients that are helping to drive the cosmetic industry today.

But how does Aloe help to keep your skin young and healthy? The answer is simple: it is known as an astringent, which simply means that it is a component that helps to tighten the tissues of your body and by increasing the elasticity of your skin. However, Aloe is also very moisturizing and hydrating, allowing your skin to feel rejuvenated in the long-term.

7. Aloe Vera Can Detoxify Your Entire Body

You may often hear how people and experts claim that you need to detoxify your body on a frequent basis just to keep it healthy and to keep your body safe from harmful bacteria and viruses that may do your body harm. But how does Aloe Vera help with detoxifying your body?

Well, Aloe is known in the medical community as a gelatinous plant food. What that means is that Aloe, very similar to seaweed, is made up a gel that when passing through your intestinal tract is able to absorb every kind of toxin it encounters along the way. This gel then pushes the toxins straight through to your colon where it will be eliminated when you have a bowel movement.

If you are looking for a way to feel healthy and want to reduce the risk of you getting sick on a frequent basis, consuming Aloe Vera often may be just the right way to go for you.

8. Aloe Vera Has The Ability To Protect You From Bacteria, Harmful Microbes, Fungi and Viruses

If you are looking to live a healthier lifestyle and want to reduce the risk of contracting all sorts of harmful bacteria, viruses, fungi and microbes, ingesting Aloe Vera on a frequent basis can help you do just that.

Just to give you an idea on what Aloe can protect you from, here is just a short list of it:

- It is considered to be a disinfectant.
- Has Anti-Fungal properties
- Has Anti-Bacterial Properties
- Is considered to be germicidal.
- Has Anti-Microbial Properties
- Can be used as an anti-biotic.
- Has Anti-Viral Properties.
- Has Anti-Septic Properties.

That is a lot of "anti's," isn't it? Aloe Vera is definitely a plant that you want to keep around the house just to have it handy in the case that you need it.

9. Aloe Is Packed Full of Amino and Fatty Acids

If you are unsure of what amino and fatty acids are, do not worry as you aren't the only one. To put it in simple terms amino acids are the building blocks of protein, which your body is made up of. Protein is one of the most basic components that you need on a daily basis just so that you can do normal everyday functions.

Likewise fatty acids are just as important as amino acids. Fatty acids are essential to sustain life. It is that simple. Without consuming fatty acids in our diet daily we can suffer extremely from it such as by developing learning disabilities, having our children develop slower than they should, suffering from many diseases that can be prevented and suffering from various skin issues.

Consuming Aloe Vera on a daily basis can help make sure that you are getting the right quantity of amino and fatty acids to help you sustain your body for the rest of your time here on this planet.

10. Aloe Can Help To Alkalize Your Body

In today's chaotic world, most of us do not really watch what we put into our systems. Sometimes we are just too busy or we tell ourselves poor nutrition is the problem of our future selves. Regardless of the reason, most often than not we are taking in too many foods that are acidic and that can do more harm to our bodies than good. While this may not seem like it is a detrimental thing to our health, it can cause a breeding ground for many diseases that can affect our health in a very negative way.

Aloe Vera is a type of plant that when it is eaten, it can help alkalize the food that you are consuming, This handy little plant can help make sure that no diseases are able to form in an environment that is very acidic and can help keep you healthy for many years to come.

As you can see there are many benefits to consuming Aloe Vera on a daily basis. Regardless of whether you decide that you want to use Aloe Vera to help you prevent a variety of potential diseases, to use it to help your skin or to help you get all the essential vitamins and minerals that you need the truth of the matter is that aloe is just all around good for your health. It is indeed a handy plant to have around your home.

Chapter Three: 8 Different Ways to Use Aloe Vera to Enhance Your Health

Whether or not you are looking for a way to keep your teeth health, to add a beautiful sheen to your hair or wanting to look younger, there are many ways that you can use Aloe Vera on a daily basis today. Some of the ways that you can put this plant to good use may surprise you in a good way. In this chapter you will learn how you can use Aloe to treat a variety of different things and learn exactly how it helps you to prevent and overcome certain health issues that you may be faced with in the future.

1. It Can Help Treat Inflammation and Wounds to Your Body

The important thing that you have to know is

that inflammation is the way that your body reacts when it gets damaged. It forces all of its energy on that one damaged area and alerts the body to send the troops in to help prevent infection. Your skin will then swell up in an effort to prevent any dangerous microbes from coming in unwanted and will then heat up in trying to kill off any dangerous organisms that may have made it passed the barrier.

So, how exactly does Aloe work to help end this natural response in your body? Aloe contains compounds in it known as plant steroids. If you are unsure of what steroids are, they have been used in both western and traditional eastern medicine to help cut the body's inflammation response in a natural way. It works by blocking the hormones that lead to the body sending out an inflammatory response.

It works to heal your body of various cuts and wounds by soothing the area with a cooling effect to help the tissues relax and the muscles to loosen around the affecting area. It will also work to fight off any bacteria or harmful microbes that try to take up residence in the wound or cut. When the aloe releases the cooling effect into your body, giving the cells in your body the opportunity to begin rebuilding the tissue that has been damaged and by creating new cells to do this.

2. Help to Treat Acne

If you are suffering from constant and annoying acne, using Aloe may be something you haven't gotten the chance to consider yet. Keep in mind though that while Aloe will never be able to complete cure you of acne, it helps to reduce the amount of redness and inflammation that you have on your face, giving you a more youthful and clear appearance.

Aloe can also help you prevent future acne outbreaks. All that you do is make a paste or gel out of the aloe and place it directly on the affected area, just like you would with any other acne medication. That's it.

3. Reduce Embarrassing Stretch Marks

Whether you have recently lost weight, gain weight or just delivered a baby, the only thing that is probably bothering you the most out of anything else on your body is perhaps the appearance of stretch marks. Having stretch marks can make you feel self-conscious to the point that even showing a touch of them will cause you to get anxious. Do not worry. You are not alone in this.

You can easily use Aloe Vera to help rid your body of bothersome stretch marks. You may have even noticed that many medications that are designed to help get rid of stretch marks contains Aloe as of the main ingredients. The truth is that Aloe can help get rid of annoying stretch marks just by simply healing the area of skin where the marks are laying.

Just make a thickened paste or gel made of Aloe Vera and apply directly on to the area where the stretch marks are. Do that on a daily basis and within a couple of weeks your stretch marks should completely disappear.

4. Help to Treat Your Loss of Hair

Losing your hair is something that many people dread. However, this is the way of life and as we age, women and men alike may begin to lose sections of their hair or may even lost the whole head of hair right off the bat. If you want to prevent this from happening to you in the future just use some Aloe.

People have used Aloe in personalized hair care treatments dating back to the ancient Egyptians. Why is that? It is simple: Aloe can help stimulate your hair to grow, even when it may not be wanting to. Even if your hair does not want to grow, Aloe can help get rid of the dead skin cells that are blocking new hair follicles from growing by eradicating them completely.

5. Help to Give Your Skin a Healthy Glow

Using Aloe Vera can help give your body the nutrients it needs to look young and healthy. As we age the cells in our skin begins to die and lose their elasticity. By using Aloe you can help rejuvenate the elasticity in your skin and to help remove the dead skin cells that are making your skin look dull.

6. Help to Ensure the Health of Your Teeth

If you are surprised to find that Aloe Vera can indeed help you to take excellent care of your teeth, do not worry. I was surprised to find this out too. However, when you make a juice using Aloe and ingest it on a frequent basis, you can help support not only perfect hygiene, but the health of your gums as well. In fact, many dentists today will recommend using Aloe especially if you have had a lot of issues with your teeth such as cavities or abscesses.

Aloe also works great for those suffering from painful dental issues such as split gums, cavities, ulcers and stomatitis in the dentures.

7. Help Alleviate Dry Skin

If you suffer from dry skin or suffer from conditions such as psoriasis or eczema, Aloe

Vera may soon become your best friend. Over many years of research, researchers have found that Aloe is very beneficial for one's skin. Due to its own moisture content, Aloe is able to moisturize your skin and make sure that your skin remains moisturized for many hours. Once you apply a generous layer over the layer of skin that is dry, the Aloe goes to work immediately releases important vitamins and minerals that will help to restore your skin's natural pH level and by applying a deep moisturizing effect to all of your tissues.

8. Get Rid of Pesky Dandruff

Anybody who has ever had dandruff knows how annoying and embarrassing it can be. Some people suffer so badly from it that they have to resort to using specially medicated shampoos. Instead of wasting money on these kinds of shampoos, simply use Aloe Vera.

Dandruff is often caused by one or two things:

1. Dead skin less on your scalp and that you have failed to shed.

2. Naturally dryness of the scalp.

So, how does Aloe work to get rid of dandruff? With its anti—fungal properties and its moisturizing ability, Aloe is able to moisturize your scalp while at the same time alleviating any itching feeling that you may be having. Use this one your scalp every day for a week or two and one day you will wake up only to suffer from dandruff no more.

There are so many uses for Aloe today that if I were to write about them all in this eBook, this book would be over one hundred pages long. There is almost no end to use of Aloe and this is the main reason it continues to be a popular plant item in most homes today. Whether you wish to treat pesky dandruff or whether you simply want to keep your skin healthy, you will not go wrong with having a pot of Aloe hanging around the house.

Conclusion

It is no secret why Aloe Vera continues to being one of the most popular plants that you will spot in anybody else's or why it continues to be used by major health and beauty companies today. Even if professionals and corporations don't truly believe that this plant has healing properties, there is certainly a reason why they insist on using or recommending it.

Research and time have shown us what Aloe is capable of doing to the human body and how it can help cure us of many common health ailments. There is no need to rely on drugs, medication or chemicals to help keep your body feeling as healthy as possible. Literally all you really need is an Aloe Vera plant somewhere in your house and you will be able to treat yourself and your family for almost any situation.

Hopefully with this eBook you have learned everything beneficial that there is to know about this plant. You have learned how this plant can help you treat common health afflictions and how it will benefit your overall health in the future. My hope is that you will soon make an Aloe Vera plant apart of your daily routine and go out to get ones of these magical plants today.

About Us

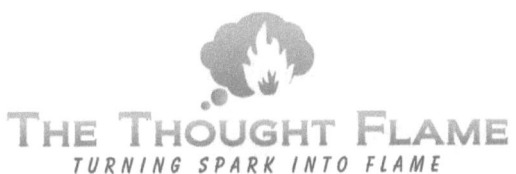

The Thought Flame is committed to add value to its customers through various books, online courses and other resources. You can learn more about us and our books at www.thethoughtflame.com.

Don't forget to check out our amazing **online video courses** at www.thethoughtflame.com/courses/ to take your knowledge to another level.

To check out our **extraordinary collection of diet/cookbooks**, visit http://www.thethoughtflame.com/category/non-fictional/cookbooks/ .

As a part of our valued relationship with our customers, we keep providing you free promotional books, courses and other stuff on subscribing with us on our site. We have a strict anti-spam policy and assure you no spam mails will be sent to your mailbox.

To subscribe with us, visit www.thethoughtflame.com.

Like our work and would like to say thanks?

Buy us a cup of coffee at www.thethoughtflame.com/coffee/

Author

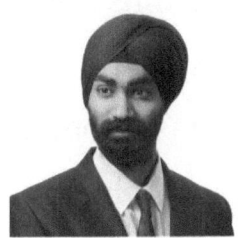

Amarpreet Singh is an avid learner and his passion for education has made him travel, work and study all across the world. He holds three masters degrees, including MBA, from top universities in Asia.

He is author of dozens of books, many of which are Amazon's bestseller, varying in various topics and categories. He also teaches many online courses having thousands of students across the world.

He has a keen interest in international affairs, economics, global poverty and politics, financial markets and entrepreneurship, and strives to be part of a community that shares the same passion.

He has worked as consultant with organizations like Airbus and The World Bank.

He loves travelling and learning about new cultures, and has been fortunate to live/work/travel/study in countries like India, China, Korea, US, South Africa, Japan, Philippines, Singapore, Canada etc., and learn about the culture and lifestyle in each of them.

To check out more of his work, visit www.thethoughtflame.com